One-Day Miracles
Change Your Brain to Master Your Weight

Michael Steven Purles
Weight-Mastery Solutions

Published by Weight-Mastery Solutions
3164 Granite Woods Lane
Sandy, UT 84092

ISBN - 10: 0615893368
ISBN - 13: 978-0615893365

:

To my wife, whose weight-mastery
journey has been inspirational

and

to all of you who desire to change your life through
mastering your weight, but haven't found a long-term
solution. This book is dedicated to you.

Table of Contents

Acknowledgements

The search to find a solution to the "yo-yo" pattern of weight loss and weight gain, that has afflicted such a large portion of our population, has been a rewarding collaborative effort.

The solution required a holistic approach, integrating the physiological processes required for good health with the actual processes required for brain and lifestyle habit change. Bringing these "points of light" together from the different areas of health science was and continues to be a very exciting journey.

This innovative and effective program could not have been accomplished without the dedicated efforts of:

- Robert B. Jones, D.C., F.A.S.A., director of the Utah Wellness Institute
- Bernell L. Christensen, Ph.D., LMFT, director of Maximum Potential
- David G. Cobb, certified fitness consultant and national trainer

This dedicated service produced the experience and understanding needed to bring this integrated, science-based program to the general public in an effective self-help format. Their contributions were invaluable.

Preface

Any self-improvement effort, whether long-term weight loss or other personal growth goal, must be developed through a process we call "dual creation." This regimen has only two steps, but each is vital and must be completed in proper order. You change or improve yourself . . .

1. First, in your mind
2. Second, in the physical world

All self-improvement occurs in your mind, in your thoughts, before you begin the physical actions that bring it about.

This book is a guide for "step one" in how to literally change your brain and your thoughts, leading to success. We have focused on weight-mastery, but the processes and tools are exactly what are needed for any self-improvement effort. The title, *One-Day Miracles, Change Your Brain to Master Your Weight*, could be *"Change Your Brain to Master Your Social Skills"* or any other goal.

Since this book is a guide for brain change, it does not include the training and recommendations for the biological requirements of optimal physical health. You won't find recipes and fitness exercises in this work. There are many sources of healthful information available to you for the second step of "dual creation."

When you have completed your study of this instruction, if you desire an integrated approach for both steps of "dual creation," we have a program that may fit your needs. The last chapter, "From Thought to Action "will provide additional information regarding it. Until then, it is time to begin to "change your brain."

Introduction

Any diet or weight loss program that does not inspire and create brain change is doomed to failure for the long term.

It has been estimated that dieters will regain two thirds of the lost weight in the first year and 95% of them will regain all of it and usually more by the end of the fifth year. Our experience with overweight and obese clients is consistent with this estimation. Perhaps this mirrors your personal experience with the "weight loss challenge."

Our clients, nearly without exception, say that they have tried everything and can't keep the lost weight from returning. They also express profound frustration with the whole matter. Some people never seem to gain weight and yet the majority of the population is overweight. Why is this so?

Well, now you know. Brain change is required to provide the enduring foundation for improved body composition, leanness, and optimal health for the long-term. It must already be in place or take place as the weight is lost.

Everything in "living your life" begins with the brain, including losing weight and keeping it off. Every action, behavior, and decision begins with a thought and is influenced by an attitude or emotion.

So, why then have researchers spent decades dealing with the physiological responses to food and behaviors and most have left the brain out of the equation? It is perplexing, because if the brain has not "bought in" or been prepared to accept the needed lifestyle changes, they won't last.

Just because you have had a thought or made a conscious decision, does not mean that your brain, as a practical matter, will go along with it. You might say, "How can that be? Am I not my brain or isn't my mind under my control?" The answer is yes . . . sort of, but only under certain conditions. Your brain operates the way it does, in part, because you have trained it to be that way.

You have influenced your brain's development and what it considers as "normal" responses to life situations by your past decisions. Some responses have become automatic, we call these habits. If you have ever tried to change a habit that has been in place for a long time, you know how difficult it is. The brain resists giving it up, requiring you to replace it in the "brain's own way."

We can tell you that most people attempt to make changes through willpower. This is not the "brain's own way." They do this rather than using the brain's process for habit creation. For this reason, they are unsuccessful.

If you haven't been able to change your habits, lifestyle, and your weight for the long-term, then you have likely missed the vital first step in the process, the rewiring of your brain to accept and facilitate the desired physiological changes. Don't underestimate the power of attitude and emotion. If they are not positive and constructive, you'll likely stay in the same mental and physical shape that you are now in.

This book was written to provide the 10 proven mental processes that you can readily make a part of your life for weight loss and long-term mastery. Each of them is vital to your success. Don't undervalue any one of them or you risk incomplete results or outright failure.

1. **Goal creation** – establish where are you going
2. **Commitment** – casual or determined?
3. **Creative visualization** – what you think about is what you do, virtual brain change
4. **Brain change** – rewiring your brain for healthy behaviors and lifestyle habit change
5. **Patience** – necessary component of personal power
6. **Willpower** – persistent use of healthy processes
7. **Give** - to create and receive a powerful, personal support structure
8. **Acquiring energy** – fill your "batteries" from all of life's sources
9. **Eliminate** - self-sabotaging thoughts
10. **Think** - like a "naturally thin" person

Remember, brain "buy-in" and preparation for lifestyle change is the necessary first step. Without it, the long-term physical changes you desire will not last. Does this make sense to you? This requirement is discussed throughout the book.

Simple, effective instruction for changes in how you see yourself and for the rewiring of your brain are the focuses of this work. If you make them, improved health and body composition will follow.

Lori's Story

Obesity was the outcome of a nearly lifelong challenge with weight management for Lori. It wasn't that she was unconcerned or had just a casual interest in taking control; she couldn't find the key to unlocking the door of long-term weight loss. She tried an untold number of diets that promised the results she longed for.

Unfortunately, the promises were never fulfilled. If she lost weight, it returned and on some diets she actually gained additional weight. Frustration and declining health became her joint companions.

Finally, the medical recommendation was made that she should have bariatric surgery. She went to a psychologist to determine if she had the mental stability to experience and profit from this extreme procedure. As she pondered what to do, she listened to her intuitive voice that questioned whether or not she could really lose the weight.

Why? Something told her that without learning to think differently about herself, food, and her eating behaviors, she would not be successful. Lori sensed that achieving her goal would require a revolutionary change in her thoughts.

Lori began searching to see if there was any program or organizational focus that aligned with her intuitive feeling. What she felt she needed was an approach or system that would assist her in true self-discovery changes.

Lori's search brought her to our program. She said that the focus and instruction lined up exactly with her needs. Lori decided she didn't require surgery. What she really needed were mental changes. This "ah ha" experience led her to understand she could take control by thinking differently. She was able to examine her true feelings about herself, life, health, food, and pleasure.

By working to change her thoughts with a new focus on what was important in her life, Lori began to eat differently. She didn't like vegetables, but even the taste of these foods became more pleasurable as brain change progressed. She began to talk about herself more positively. Food stopped being her "best friend" and became the fuel for energy. Her health improved and she now does not need bariatric surgery. Brain and thought change delivered the desired results.

A Warning

Many people wish they could take a pill and long-term weight loss would be theirs. In today's culture, we often want immediate results with little effort. It would be wonderful if weight-mastery could be delivered like this, but it cannot. It is impossible for any pill, product or "revolutionary" aid to deliver long-term results.

Most diet and weight loss programs do not provide the processes and tools required for brain change. Changes of habits and lifestyle must be made in the brain's own way.

You've probably discovered that willpower does not create brain change. Weight-mastery and optimal health are the end result of healthful adjustments to a person's (1) thoughts and (2) actions, (3) applied over time with consistency.

Let's say that again with different words. Long-term weight management requires managed changes of thought and action, which produce a rewiring of your brain with new, healthy default habits. *One-Day Miracles* provides the processes and mental tools for thought change, so that your actions will deliver the desired results.

One-Day Miracles

You've had difficult challenges in your life as we all have. Basic human experience, evidenced and shared throughout history, verifies that we all have the ability to meet even difficult challenges for one single day. Great accomplishments are made in single days.

Sometimes small, incremental, daily steps are the vital actions preceding the performing of a miracle. These steps are always designed and launched by our thoughts.

Healthy physical actions or strategies (like exercise or consuming healthy foods), when combined with the rewiring of your brain will provide results that can be felt, seen, and made a record of on a daily basis. In fact, we encourage you to keep a journal and write in it daily, but more will be said on this later.

In fact, single days have proved to be marvelous, even magical, points in time that have brought wonderful rewards to you. On one day you were born, graduated from school, got a job, got married, and won the lottery.

OK, maybe you didn't do all of these, but think about the miracles that occurred on one day in your life. Now, we know that other productive days may have been required to get to these days, but that is the miracle of it all. Stringing single, focused days together creates miracles of blessing in our individual lives.

One single day in the 30,000 days of your life can make all the difference for your health and wellbeing—the one day you didn't think you could handle, but you did and everything changed. It is amazing what a person can accomplish (or endure) within a single day to bless their lives. If you are prepared, "today" will be replicated for the next day and the next, until your goal of weight-mastery is achieved. There are "one-day miracles" ahead of you now. Enjoy and revel in them.

Daily To-Do List

Becoming organized and consistent in the use of the mental processes and tools detailed here is vital to your success. This effort will take some time and organization. A simple daily "to-do" list can become one of your most powerful tools if you will invest yourself in it. It doesn't matter if it is on paper, computer, or smartphone. It needs to be recorded where you will see it at the beginning of and throughout each day as needed.

What? You don't use a to-do or check-off list? Well, this needs to become your first new healthy habit. Make a "to-do list" a part of your daily regimen until your brain accepts it as a default (pre-programmed) behavior. Our suggested list will be shared with you at the end of the book. Don't wait until you come to that to get started. From what you have learned in this chapter, are there some daily things you should be doing right now? Make a list of them here.

_____

_____

_____

_____

_____

_____

_____

_____

_____

_____

Important Information

> Before engaging in any weight loss diet or program, including the recommendations and tools offered in this book, you should be examined by your healthcare practitioner to determine if you are physically and mentally healthy enough to participate in a weight loss program that may include: changes in your diet, an exercise regimen, supplementation, and other tools. The processes and tools offered here may not be appropriate for all health and physical situations.

Your Thoughts:

(Wherever you see this subtitle, take a few minutes and write down your thoughts and impressions about the instruction and "you" in the space provided. Personalize this book to meet your needs in the way that you learn so that you can come to "own" the material and processes, and make them work for you.)

Goals and Commitment

". . . in order to change your body, you must first change your brain." Daniel G. Amen, MD, neuroscientist and brain imaging expert

"You can't tell where you are in life until you know where you are going." Where you are right now is always in relationship to where you want to be. So, you've decided you need to master your weight by rewiring your brain and changing the way that you think. We cheer you on, but what does that mean to you? Can you identify specifically the outcomes you want to achieve? You can, good! Get them in writing. It has been said that a goal that is not written is really only a wish.

For you to be successful, your goals, expectations, and efforts must be clearly determined and prioritized. Are they worth living and working for? If not, it is easy to abandon them when you've had a bad week or things are more difficult than you had anticipated.

When challenging times come (and they will — you know that) you need the support of clearly identified goals that mean more to you than the "price" that needs to be paid to achieve them. They need to be prioritized and written down.

The method or document that we recommend is a self-contract. This is an effective tool to keep you focused and progressing on your weight loss and health goals. It may be the "deciding factor" in your drive to become the master of your weight. More will be explained regarding this document.

"Anti-Goal" List

This may seem a little strange to you, but thoughtfully prepare a list of the attitudes and behaviors that you want to get rid of, an "anti-goal list." This becomes a record comprised of your current unhealthy behaviors and attitudes that you want replaced.

Tag this as your "garbage" list, the items you want taken out to the trash and disposed of. The only way this can happen is to replace them with new healthy attitudes and behaviors. Be honest and use the list to measure your progress in replacing each of your health compromising practices.

Your list might include things like:

- Emotional eating
- Skipping meals like breakfast
- Desserts after lunch and dinner
- Eating too many carbohydrates, lots of sugar
- Eating too many prepared foods
- Too few vegetables
- Over-eating
- Getting popcorn and a soda at the movies
- Getting a candy bar when I get gas

- Eating too fast
- I'm too weak, no will power
- I'm afraid of success
- Lots of negative thoughts and attitudes

"Replacement" Goals

Take a few minutes to think through your desires and write down your health goals. Use a pencil at first so you can make changes. When you think the list is complete, set it aside. Let your mind and heart continue to ponder what has been written and what has not for a while.

After a few hours, perhaps even over night, review the list once again and make any necessary changes. Then, if you are convinced that this is what you want to accomplish, it is time to put together a "self-contract."

On the top of a sheet of paper type or write: "My Weight Loss and Health Goals Contract." In priority order, list each of the goals, being specific about what you want to accomplish. If the goal is a large one or has different steps needed for accomplishment, break it down into smaller (bite size) goals that are more easily managed.

Can each of the goals be measured? Can you tell when you have achieved them? Are there reasonable dates for fulfillment? If so, list them along with the goal. Answers to all of these questions are important.

Then, this language is vital. Under the goals, write: "I hereby agree and commit to achieve these goals and gain long-term control of my weight and health." Sign your name and the date under this commitment. Now you have a contract with yourself. Are you determined to honor it? Don't give yourself a pass on this. The contract has incredible value. It is another tool in your hand to keep your progressing.

There is one more thing. These goals need to be shared with at least one other trustworthy person, who will actively support you in achieving them. We call this person a "Support Partner" and more of her or his potential help will be discussed in the chapter titled "Give to Receive." This person should sign below your signature and be given a copy of the contract.

Keep a copy in front of you throughout the process as a constant reminder of your priorities and commitment to achieve them. This will be especially helpful on bad days and times when you may be tempted to give up. Bad moments and difficult periods will come, but if you stay focused they'll disappear and you'll be stronger than ever. Don't take any chances. Keep this and other motivational reminders in front of you. Don't be afraid to add or subtract goals as your life progresses.

Now that you know the process, here are some target areas that you may find appropriate to specifically identify the results that you want to achieve.

- Clothes sizes
  - Dress
  - Shirt
  - Jacket
  - Pants
- Body dimensions
  - Neck
  - Upper arms
  - Chest
  - Waist
  - Thighs
- % Body fat (you can use the Body Mass Index, BMI, or specialized body fat measuring tools)

Tracking and validating your progress from day to day will be discussed in the chapter on "Patience and Validation."

Commitment

Your answer to this question is vital to your success. "How committed are you to changing your life and improving your health?" The follow-up question is just as important, "Are you willing to follow a plan (carefully prepared by you), one that does not require difficult tasks, but does require consistency and repetition, until you have reached your goal? We hope both of your answers are an emphatic "yes." If your interest is only casual, then your responses and effort will be the same—insufficient to attain your goal.

Your Thoughts:

Dual Creation

"If you think you can do a thing or think you can't do a thing, you're right." Henry Ford

What you think about is what you do. This is especially true regarding your perceptions about you. By the way, researchers tell us that our perceptions of things (even if they are wrong) constitute about 90% of our reality.

What are your thoughts or perceptions about you? Are you weak, a loser, undeserving of life's good things, and stuck with ill health and a body that refuses to release weight?

Perhaps your perceptions are that you are a person of value, possessing talents, energy, power, and the ability to change your body and life for the better.

How you see yourself, really see yourself, is essential to mastering your weight and changing your life. If you can't believe that you can do it, then failure will be the outcome, because you have already predetermined it. But know this, if that is the way you feel now, you can change it. Perceptions and their attendant thoughts don't have to be set in stone, immovable, and unchangeable.

You can change all of that! You must change all of it!

Losing weight and keeping it off begin in your mind — some might say that this is in a real way "thinking yourself to become thin." To create the new slimmer, healthier you, you must reconstruct yourself:

1. First in your mind
2. Then, in the physical world

This new vision, comprised of the right thoughts, is absolutely necessary for the physical manifestation to take place.

Stop thinking like an overweight person and start thinking like a lean or thin person. This is the necessary first step to behaving like one.

Lynn's Story

Lynn had been of normal weight most of her life. She tried to eat responsibly and enjoyed physical activity, but was not a devoted exerciser. Her weight began to creep up over time and soon she jumped three dress sizes. When she looked in the mirror, she didn't like what she saw.

Following traditional lines of weight loss thinking, she reduced her daily calorie load, continued eating responsibly, and began getting significant exercise at least three days a week. She even joined a health club. After two years she had lost only two pounds.

You probably understand how discouraged and frustrated she felt. After all of that effort and time, there was certainly a temptation to say, "I've done all I can and I guess this is who I am. I'm going to just have to live with it."

Lynn didn't do that. In fact, even after what felt like complete failure, she continued to think about herself as a lean or thin individual. Lynn said she never gave into the thought that she had to think of herself as a heavy person.

In her mind's eye she still had a lean body composition.

This self-perception was the core component for turning her situation around. You probably want to know the outcome — well, she figured out what her body's needs were, because she didn't permit her thoughts to change from being a lean and healthy person. She dropped the three dress sizes and has kept the weight off long-term.

Creative Visualization

The technique of using one's mind or imagination to form a mental image of behaviors or life events is called creative visualization. It can play a significant role in successful outcomes in your life, including establishing different lifestyle behaviors for losing weight, keeping it off, and improving your health.

This technique has undergone significant scientific research as well as practical application by very successful people such as: Tiger Woods (golf), Anthony Robbins (peak performance strategist), Bill Gates (Microsoft cofounder), Will Smith (actor), and many others in music and other life endeavors.

A very famous study was conducted at the Harvard Medical School by neuroscientist Alvaro Pascual-Leone. He had two groups of volunteers perform a simple exercise by two different methods to determine the effects on the brain.

The first group learned and practiced a five-finger piano exercise for two hours a day for five days, trying to keep the metronome at 60 beats per minute. At the end of the trial, scientific measurements were taken of the affected areas of the brain.

It was found that an expansion or reorganization of the cortex (outermost layer) of the brain had taken place to accommodate what had been practiced and learned. The brain had created a direct tissue response to the physical activity of playing this piano exercise.

Alvaro Pascual-Leone said that the second group, "instead of practicing at the keyboard two hours daily for five days, spent time at the keyboard visualizing, rather than executing, the movements."

This second group never actually played the piano, except in their heads as they visualized their fingers touching each key in the proper order. Brain scans of this group showed similar levels of brain change as that experienced by the physical practice group!

This is important to understand. Thinking about the exercise pattern and the individual movement of fingers, produced the same kind of brain change in the second group as physically moving them did for the first group.

Well, what does that have to do with achieving weight-mastery? Everything! It becomes obvious from this experiment and many others like it that the brain can't tell the difference between a "real" experience and a visualized one. You can use this tremendous brain attribute to your advantage by visualizing the behaviors that will improve your health.

To get the right outcome from creative visualization, it must be done on a daily basis in order for actual brain change to take place. Begin this mental exercise tomorrow to master your weight. Spend five minutes, right after waking in the morning, visualizing yourself as a lean or thin person and the "thin" behaviors you will employ throughout the day.

Pick a spot that is quiet, comfortable, and where you can close your eyes. Visualize yourself thin and in control. Visualize each of the meals/snacks and behaviors that will be a part of your day. See yourself in control and experience how you will feel without those extra pounds.

Encourage the positive emotions that are a natural outcome of the anticipation of goal achievement to fill you mind and your body. Let them work through you until you nearly tingle from the excitement of being the master of your weight. Revel in the pleasure and wellbeing you're experiencing. Let the "high" strengthen your commitment to continue working and become the person you are envisioning. Feel it! Embrace it! Become it!

What if you are not able to experience this life-changing "high" right away? Don't become discouraged. Keep at it. Your brain has to be trained to think and perceive in new ways. You've spent many years training it to respond as it does now, so some adaptation time is expected.

Now, you are going to retrain your mind in a positive way to support your goals and that may take some time. Remember, visualization must be done each day. Don't stop because you haven't experienced the "high" yet, or because you have and you feel like you've arrived. It may take months of using this simple exercise to help you achieve your goal, but it is powerful when used consistently over time.

Your Thoughts:

"I Don't Have to Do That"

"Cut the mental fat, and that will lead to cutting the waistline fat." Pamela Peeke, MD

Why is long-term success so hard to achieve? Nearly every reputable plan and program works on reducing the consumption of calories and/or a plan for burning them. If you consume fewer calories than you need, you lose weight. If you consume more than you need, you gain weight. There is no other way around it. This is a universal truth, even though there are individual differences in body chemistry and the rate of calorie burning.

How you facilitate the consumption and burning — the kinds of decisions that you make are governed by your brain. There are additional contributing factors that may help or hurt, but that is the bottom line. Your brain is the key.

Acquiring long-term mastery of your weight requires you to change those behaviors and habits that have a negative impact. This means a change in the way your brain is "wired."

Long time habits have deep and strong neural pathways. These must be encouraged to shrink and weaken from disuse, while the pathways of the new, healthy habits are being strengthened and deepened.

You know that you need to change your dietary habits and your lifestyle. You've probably tried many times, making resolutions and beginning the effort, but the outcome is always the same. Why? Perhaps you've become convinced that you do not have the necessary willpower; after all that's what others may have suggested and perhaps you've concluded that yourself. <u>This is absolutely not true!</u>

Brain change cannot be done by the exercise of willpower alone (more will be said on the role of willpower later). It must be done in the brain's own way. This is what you will learn in this chapter.

You have natural strengths that are working against you — your brain's habit-forming abilities. What you may not realize is that the resolution of your weight loss concerns is already built into the structure and operation of your brain. Learning how to use your brain's control in habit formation and decision-making will give you the power to achieve your weight-mastery goals.

Habits and Decision-Making

Your brain is so complex and sophisticated that its functions cannot be duplicated. With over 100 billion neurons, making over 100 trillion connections, brain events occur in fractions of milliseconds or over longer periods of time, according to need.

With efficiency being the brain's number one goal, habit formation is the number one priority to meet that goal. Think about it. If you had to look at instructions every morning on how to tie your shoes, start the car, or drive to work, how efficient would you be? As you can see, habits are incredibly beneficial — most of the time.

Habits require the investment of time, repetition, and energy. As a result, your brain doesn't want to give them up. In fact, it is structured to hang on to them, irrespective of whether they are ultimately healthy or unhealthy. The brain constitutes only about 2% of your body's weight and uses about 25% of the calories you consume. Efficiency is vital to your wellbeing.

Over your lifetime, you have developed the habits that have contributed to your weight problem. Think back on some of your past eating decisions (adventures) or ones that confront you now on a regular basis. Have you made the unhealthy choice, even though you know better? Have you let unhealthy urges or cravings direct your choices? Why do you keep making the bad choice when reason tells you to make the right one?

Don't even begin to think that you are not strong enough. That isn't the cause. Centered in your brain is a "decision-making system" that is involved in every choice you make. Its operation has been preprogrammed somewhat by earlier repetitive decisions you have made.

To overcome unhealthy and unwelcome behaviors you need to learn how this decision system works, so that you can direct it to make the choices you want most. When directing it with the tools and methods you will learn in this book, you will chart new paths of behavior that will positively affect every aspect of your life.

Forming Habits is the Brain's #1 Priority

Making a decision does not generate a habit. They require the growth of neural pathways, using time and repetition to create them. When behaviors are repeated frequently, strong neural pathways are developed and your responses become routine to certain repetitive situations. When this happens the brain moves these "automatic responses" into the subconscious as habits.

Think about your own history of habit formation. How long did it take you to learn to habitually wear a seatbelt, especially if you went a long time beforehand without buckling up? Creating the habit required the investment of time, focus, energy, physical movement, and repetition. Habits free the brain up to focus on other activities and skills. This is how we continue to grow. Without habits we couldn't get very far in life.

The brain does not evaluate within the habit-forming process whether or not the habit is good or bad, healthy or unhealthy. Your brain has invested a great deal of time, perhaps years, and effort in learning the techniques and details of a habit or behavior. Can you see why it guards them so jealously and doesn't want to give them up?

Remember, the brain wants to be efficient. Giving up a habit means wasting years of effort, energy and learning — something inefficient to the brain.

Can It Be Done?

Does this mean that you're stuck with your current habits? No! Can a habit or behavior be changed? Absolutely! The requirement is to acquire the appropriate knowledge and tools, and then supply consistent practice to replace the old habit with a new one. The initial step is to understand how habits are developed, even the negative ones. This knowledge will permit you to take charge and make the changes you desire.

Our brains have two powerful centers that can become conflicted about how a decision should be made — one is logical and reasoning, the other emotional and reactive. For our purposes and the ease of using a characterization we are all familiar with, we'll call the logical center the "Angel" and the emotional center the "Devil." Besides, you may find some comfort in saying, "The Devil made me do it."

It is important to understand that each center is vital to your mental health, each having attributes needed by you at different times and in different situations. Decisions are not necessarily made by these centers — they work powerfully to influence them. You, your conscious mind, makes the final decision, unless you let habits become the "default decision maker."

Take some time and try to visualize these two powerful influencers making your decisions for you. You have had decisions to make when strong emotion pulled you one way and logical reasoning presented a different path. Perhaps you have felt at those times that you are two different people, one logical and in control, and the other emotional and sometimes out of control. Let's take a look at each of these decision influencers.

Angel: this is the brain area known as the prefrontal cortex, the first 1/3 of your brain. It acts like a supervisor, involved in attention or focus, logic, judgment, decision-making, planning, and impulse control. Its attributes are the ones that fill you with confidence that you are headed in the right direction and you can proceed positively under its direction.

When following the "Angel's" guidance in decision-making you might hear, "I've considered the healthiest approach to resolve this feeling of intense stress and I think taking a peaceful walk after work is best."

Devil: the deep limbic system lies near the center of the brain, encompassing several structures. This is the area that sets a person's emotional tone. This part of your mind can be loud, reactive, and highly dramatic, demanding its own way "right now!" It also can make you aware of your most powerful feelings and emotions like fear, craving, depression, anger, and many positive, self-protecting emotions as well.

As a participant in decision-making, the "Devil" might say, "Listen up, I'm craving some relief and I don't think a walk will do it. I want relief right now! I want a candy bar and I'm not going to wait! "

The Negative Habits "Script"

Based upon previous experience and repetitive decisions made, the Angel (logic) and Devil (emotion) may interact in a scripted or predictive manner that produces and reinforces negative habits and behaviors. Focus on this example:

You are driving home after a difficult day at work and your Devil takes center stage in your mind screaming, "I'm stressed! I need something to make me feel better and I need it right now!"

The Angel may try to get control of the situation by

suggesting a healthy and logical approach such as, "We'll go for a long walk when we get home and you'll feel much better."

The Devil refuses to go along. A remedy is suggested. "Based on previous choices, the cure at the top of the list for this kind of stress, the thing that will give immediate relief and pleasure is a milkshake and fries." The Devil says, "That's what we've always done and that's what I want. We'll focus on that right now."

"There's a fast-food place on the way home. Here are the directions to get there." A solution and plan has been suggested, one that has been repeated many times before.

The Devil will not take "no" for an answer and refuses to let the Angel take control of the situation. It says, "I'm stressed out of my mind. A milkshake and fries are at the top of the list and we have a plan to get to a fast-food restaurant immediately. This is what we're going to do and I won't take no for an answer!"

The intense emotion and impulsive demand finally convinces the Angel to surrender. It follows the Devil's orders, giving up its natural role as a powerful, controlled, and logical leader. It then uses its ability to create focus without distraction on getting to the fast-food restaurant.

When the Angel "buys" in to this resolve, any other thoughts such as, "You don't really need that kind of food. You know you'll regret it later," are quickly blocked by it.

The imperative focus is on getting to the restaurant, while all other warnings are ignored.

The route to get there is firmly planted in your mind. In fact, you visualize yourself walking in and where you will sit. The experience unfolds in greater detail as you can almost taste the food, knowing what you will order. The craving takes over with the Devil in full control.

You arrive at the restaurant and your visualization is fulfilled. As you drive home the craving disappears, leaving you feeling different – temporarily satisfied. The Angel is now left alone and earlier thoughts of reason and self-control return. Finally, with all the intense emotion drained away, you ask yourself in frustration, "Why did I give in, again? What was I thinking?"

Guess what? From a brain science point of view, you weren't thinking, at least not clearly. In fact, you couldn't! With the Devil's domination and dictation of the script to be followed, getting the fast food was the predictable outcome. Remember, this all occurred because this resolve was the one repeated so often in prior, similar experiences that it has become the priority resolution—essentially a habit. Consider your own life. You've had experiences like this, haven't you?

"Feel Good" Brain Chemicals

When your Devil screams insistently for something

that feels good, it is, in fact, a demand for an increase in the brain chemical principally responsible for feelings of well-being and pleasure. This chemical is dopamine. When your Angel gives in to these urges for unhealthy food or over eating, you are actually self-medicating to cause a release of dopamine.

Dopamine release can be caused from drugs, such as cocaine and alcohol, foods, exercise, sex, and other behaviors. Self-medication can become an addictive act with the end goal to increase those feelings of well-being and pleasure. When food is the "drug of choice," is it green vegetables that people choose or is it high calorie foods loaded with carbohydrates (sugars) and fats? Can you see the challenge here? Having enough dopamine in our lives is important, so is causing its release in appropriate ways. Healthy alternatives will be discussed in this chapter.

If this unhealthy behavior has become a habit and is the desired response for "triggering situations" (as in the previous example), there is addiction on two levels: (1) in the brain with the habit itself and (2) physiologically from dopamine's effects.

This is a good time to make a list of your unhealthy eating habits and foods so that you can focus on developing new healthy behaviors and habits to replace them.

_____

_____

_____

_____

_____

_____

_____

_____

_____

_____

Who Is In Charge?

The brain's intent, regarding habits, is to make the logical and emotional brain centers follow the same "automatic," time-tested script in responding to similar situations. You end up responding or reacting the same way each time. The brain's effort to do this is not good or bad. As you can see, everything depends on how it is used.

In a negative habit or addiction the roles of the Angel and Devil end up being the same each time.

1. The Devil comes onto the theater of the mind demanding attention and relief.
2. The prioritized and most often used solution is demanded.
3. The steps to make it occur are outlined.
4. The Angel surrenders to the Devil's demands, giving up its power, and consents to facilitating the behavior and resolve.

In these negative script situations, the Devil often ends up being in charge concerning negative habits, behaviors, and addictions.

Negative Habit Interventions

The most effective manner to convince the brain that new, healthy habits are needed is to confront it with the truth about why the old ones are unhealthy and harmful. Simultaneous with the confrontation is the active application of the new habits as replacements, being consistent over time with their use. Be advised, because your brain does not want to give up the old habits, it will take some time, perhaps months, before the new ones become "automatic." So, don't give up, because this part of brain change doesn't happen quickly.

This simple tool will allow you to put your Angel in charge. Your logical self will have a new set of operational orders and scripts to replace the old ones. New healthy behaviors will be the result. When these become your automatic defaults, you will have attained a vital step in weight-mastery.

Having a powerful decision-making influence (your Devil) that operates on emotion is a little like having an unruly child, one that always seeks attention. If you were instructing a small group of children and one of them kept talking out, disrupting, and demanding, how would you handle it? What would the likely outcome be if you do nothing?

In all likelihood you probably would follow this intervention pattern:

- Explain to the child why his or her attitude and behavior isn't proper or healthy
- Detail what the proper attitude and behavior is
- Consistently intervene every time the inappropriate behavior is exhibited
- Continue until the instruction has been internalized and the behavior has changed

You must consider the Devil's emotional influence in your decision-making process to be very similar to the "unruly child's" demands. The process of creating brain change — decision-making change, is much the same. Young and old brains respond positively to this interventional process.

Self-Talk

Food cravings and the flooding of your mind with thoughts about food are clear signals that your Devil is trying to exert control. You can put your Angel in charge. To do this you need operating orders for new habits that reflect <u>truth</u> and your healthy desires.

These new orders will be written into a script form, as if you were presenting them to another person. (That is not so far-fetched when you consider how difficult it is to access your subconscious mind.) They will be used to replace the old orders and habits that you've been automatically following.

Understanding the role of "triggers" and your responses is vitally important to good health and this process. An example of a trigger is the smell of fresh popcorn. It may initiate an urge to eat a bowl full, even though your sense of hunger had previously been satisfied.

A trigger is anything that inspires or initiates a habitual reaction and it can be positive or negative in nature. For our purposes we will only focus on negative behavior responses.

Triggers can be almost anything from an external stimulus to an internal emotion. Without intervention, they may become the instigators of unhealthy consequences.

❑ **Visual and Sensory Stimulation** — includes any type of an advertisement, whether printed,

TV, radio, or Internet that stimulates you into an unwanted and unhealthy eating behavior. It includes smells, sounds, and situations like walking by a shop window, smelling popcorn, or seeing someone eating a food that triggers the same urge.

❏ **Meal Delay** — skipping a meal or going too long between meals.

❏ **Social (eating with others)** — someone who sabotages your situation by bringing you food that is unhealthy, at a time that you don't need it, or entices you to join him in an unwanted eating behavior. It also includes consuming more than is needful, because of the social situation.

❏ **Habitual eating** — eating when there is a break in activity (boredom), eating the same food at the same time each day when it's not needed, or eating food that is associated with another activity like consuming a large soda when watching a movie, or buying a candy bar whenever you fill the car with gasoline.

❏ **Emotional** — feeling bored or burned out, lonely, angry, apathetic or afraid, stressed, or tired.

Take a few minutes and think about the different triggers for unhealthy eating behaviors that you experience. Make a list of them, including the habitual response behavior that follows. You are going to need this as you plan and program your mind to take you in a new healthy direction.

_____

_____

_____

_____

_____

_____

_____

_____

Now comes the "self-talk." Knowing what your triggers are, you can plan, practice, and prepare the interventions that will help your brain let go of the unhealthy "default" habits. You will replace them with new healthy ones of your choosing.

There are four simple steps to Self-Talk:

1. When you experience a trigger and begin to feel the urge to perform an unhealthy behavior, say to yourself, **"I don't have to do that."** Say it with emotion and out loud if you can. This will cause a momentary pause in the pressure of the urge to permit your Angel to take control.

2. Follow this emotional declaration with a quick recital of the negative urge and its unhealthy consequences. For example: "Eating a candy bar will only make me feel better for a few minutes and I'll gain weight, lose energy, and feel crummy. It's not worth it!"

3. Then, declare what your new behavior is and its benefits: "I'm not going to do that. Instead, I'm going to eat a healthy snack. I've lost weight, gained energy, and I'm happy and feeling wonderful." Say this as if you are already doing it. The brain responds with greater power and energy to positive statements.

4. Once you have explored and experimented with Self-Talk, write down this new healthy script and learn it. You need to know it, not necessarily word perfect, but as to the important points. If you have triggers that require different replacements, you might need a second healthy script. Learn them both.

Using the urge to eat a candy bar as an example, here is how Self-Talk is used:

1. "I don't have to do that."

2. "Eating a candy bar will only make me feel better for a few minutes and I'll gain weight, lose energy, and feel crummy. It's not worth it."

3. "I'm not going to do that. Instead, I'm going to eat a healthy snack. I've lost weight, gained energy, and I'm happy and feeling wonderful."

Do you recognize all the emotion and positive attributes used in this example? It is short and sweet, but has all the elements needed for you to take control.

There is any number of replacement behaviors that you might use. Here are some suggestions to get you thinking:

• Eat a healthy snack	• Call my best friend
• Go for a walk or run	• Exercise
• Work on my hobby	• Assemble a jigsaw puzzle
• Set a date for a fun activity	• Write in my journal
• Read a book or magazine article	• Practice a new skill

As you can see, the replacement doesn't have to be an eating behavior. It can be something else that requires your attention, and is healthy and pleasurable. If you are truly hungry, keep healthy snacks available as a replacement.

Practice

As you will recall from your reading on visualization, the brain can't tell the difference from a visualized experience and a real one. So, why not take advantage of this mental attribute? Take yourself through daily, visualized Self-Talk experiences to make you stronger and to accelerate the rewiring of your brain before an unhealthy urge strikes? This is the smart and healthy thing to do.

It won't take much time for you to learn how to use the Self-Talk process to assist in rewiring your brain. We recommend five minutes in the morning and evening, until it becomes natural for you to intervene whenever you feel an unhealthy urge.

What about Setbacks or Interruptions?

What if you are overcome by a craving or urge, and you end up giving in? The direct answer is, "Get over it!" You haven't failed. Just reset what you are doing, keep going, and stop worrying about it.

We cannot always dictate the environment we would like around us. Consider the challenge of your boss's invitation for dessert after the ball game or some other "pressure" situation. If you have a setback, it is OK! Your quest has not been derailed or ruined. Pick yourself up and start again. This is a necessary part of life.

As you improve in one area, you can begin focusing on another. Set yourself up for success. For example, you might begin with "eating much more at a meal than you need," and once that behavior is under control, consider adding another. It's extremely important to start with reasonable goals and slowly progress from one level to the next. Remember, it takes time and repetition for the brain to lay down new neural pathways and habits, while shrinking old unwanted behavior circuitry.

At the beginning or end of each day, as part of your daily routine, go to your journal and record your setbacks and successes. Describe how they felt and how you can capitalize on what you have learned. Make writing a "Daily Goal."

Your Thoughts:

The Role of Willpower

"The more things you do, the more you can do."
Lucille Ball

"You are the only person on earth who can use your ability." Zig Ziglar

These quotes begin to address the real role of willpower in changing your life and mastering your weight. Unfortunately, willpower is often misunderstood and misused in making life changes, especially regarding habits. The definition and effective use of "willpower" will be developed throughout this chapter.

Perhaps you've become convinced that you do not have the necessary willpower to change your life. After all, that's what others may have suggested as well. <u>This is absolutely not true!</u>

What Do You Believe About You?

If you're struggling with your weight, then you probably have unhealthy eating behaviors — not because you're weak, a failure, or lack willpower — but because you have powerful strengths that have been working against you. Coming to understand how these so-called weaknesses can become strengths will be your first task.

As you start to examine the underlying causes or

reasons for your weight-gaining behaviors, it's very important to identify certain "untruths" that you may currently believe about yourself. These barriers have to be eliminated, because they are <u>not</u> true. To make the mental changes needed for weight-mastery, you must be dealing with the truth.

1. "Because I am overweight I must not have the self-control or abilities that others have."

   This challenge with your weight has nothing to do with your innate worth or self-control (willpower). You have enormous value and potential! You simply need the right knowledge, tools, skills, and practice to change over time. As you do, your self-esteem and confidence will grow.

2. "I've tried to break free of this many times. My successes have always been temporary. I guess I just can't do it."

   There are many ways to lose weight, but as you have learned, for you they only work temporarily. Brain change is the missing requirement that was not available in the other programs and processes you've tried.

3. "You're just not trying hard enough! If you were more determined you could overcome this. If you really wanted it badly enough, you would do it."

None of these statements are true, nor are they helpful. In fact, this approach may be a big part of the reason you've been unsuccessful. More willpower is not the answer.

Doing battle in your mind to keep out thoughts about food or triggers that invite negative eating behaviors only makes the problem worse. **A different approach than you've used in the past is needed – one based on true and effective principles of change;** one that focuses on healthy eating choices; one that will literally build new brain circuitry that no longer defaults to unhealthy eating behaviors.

Willpower Is an Ineffective Shortcut Solution

When the urge arises for you to engage in a negative behavior, what is your usual response? Isn't it to exert your will and put the thought out of your mind? How successful are you? You've found it to be very difficult to do – the act seems to intensify the urge until it is almost overpowering.

When attempting to exercise willpower over an unwanted thought, craving, or urge, you are actually trying to prevent your "Devil" from taking over and demanding an unhealthy behavior. There is danger here, because attempting to exercise "sheer determination" can plunge a person into what is called the "Avoidance Cycle."

Let's go back and examine our milkshake and fries example from the "I Don't Have to Do That" chapter to understand what happens in the Avoidance Cycle.

Once again you've had a stressful day and your emotional

*self demands relief, something that feels good. A milkshake
and fries are the priority resolve from prior experience. A
plan is quickly provided to get to a favorite fast-food
restaurant. Your Angel resists and attempts to dismiss the
idea with a replacement resolve. Remember, your Angel is
responsible for logic, reasoning, and weighing options. It
sees that this is not the right decision, but the pressure from
the Devil continues to mount until the Angel finally gives
in.*

*After the event is over and the Angel is alone, it then
contemplates what occurred and wonders why it gave in
and why it always gives in. After the fact, you feel guilty.
You make the pledge that this is the last time this will
happen. You're going to take control once and for all!*

When the urge hits once again, the process plays out
one more time in the same way: (1) resisting, (2)
giving in, (3) feeling regret, and (4) committing to try
harder. Over time you eventually stop fighting the
urge and just give in. Giving in becomes the desirable
option over the depressing cycle of resisting, fighting,
giving in anyway, and then feeling guilty. As you can
see, sheer willpower is not the answer.

If using willpower in this way is not the answer, what
is? Your own natural ability to change your brain
pathways is the answer.

Why fight against the brain's natural tendency?
Change the brain's "wiring" using its own tools and

processes for habit formation. Shrink unwanted pathways and delete the negative scripts your logical and emotional brain centers are following. Give them new desirable scripts to follow using the proven principles and tools you are being taught.

Positive, permanent change will be the result. As you follow new scripts, the neural pathways for the old will diminish in influence and size over time. If you provide enough visualized and actual use practice, the neural pathways of the new, healthy habits will grow sufficiently strong enough to become the default or "automatic" habits and behaviors that you desire. The negative scripts will disappear, and a new age of brain and body health will arrive.

What Is the Role of Willpower?

It is very simple — persistency. Let's say it in another way: you are determined, relentless, and constant in the use of life changing tools. It means you don't quit. You stay at the process until the goal has been reached, utilizing your own natural strengths and abilities.

Trying to make willpower the "process" alone is a losing battle. So, now that you know all about how brains and habits are changed, make up your mind to be persistent, determined, relentless, and constant until you have acquired the "prize."

Your Thoughts:

Patience and Validation

"All human power is a compound of time and patience." Honore de Balzac

A man who is a master of patience is master of everything else. George Savile

Patience is such an interesting human quality. Most of us say we don't have enough of it and yet we must exercise it to achieve the success we desire.

In this work's introduction, the value, desirability, and necessity of obtaining "one-day miracles" were discussed. Accepting that they have value for you suggests that "patience" must be your companion to obtain them. "One-day miracles" are the positive expressions of patience.

Obtaining weight-mastery is not an event. It is a process and one that will not come to fulfillment in a day, a week, or even a month. How are you going to deal with that?

Keep your focus and expectation, not on the anxiety of reaching your goal, but on the beauty and power of achieving small measurable steps, "one-day miracles," until you have arrived.

Validation

Knowing that you are making progress makes it easier to be patient in achieving your desired outcomes. Your "self-contract" is a valuable tool in this regard.

You have completed "My Weight Loss and Health Goals Contract" haven't you? It is the blueprint for success and you need to know if you are making progress with each of the individual goals.

If you haven't, well, consider this the poke you need to get it done. Stop here and go back to the "Goals and Commitment" chapter. Spend the effort necessary. It will pay more dividends than you can imagine.

Here is something to think about as you consider the importance of weight loss. This book has as its strategic focus the necessity of brain change and reordering your thoughts for long-term weight loss. As you begin performing healthier behaviors, which should include daily physical activity, you may not lose as much weight as you originally anticipated and yet you are experiencing important success.

Here's why. Physical activity helps to increase muscle mass as fat mass decreases. Muscle weighs more than fat. As a result you may very well lose inches, but not as much weight as you thought. You women: if you dropped three to four dress sizes, but not as much weight as was your goal, would you be unhappy?

We guess probably not. There are many components

to long-term weight loss and optimal health. Changing your body composition from fat to muscle is one of them. By the way, muscle burns calories and fat does not. Increasing muscle mass will help you burn more calories on a daily basis.

Tracking your goals and targets frequently is vital to maintaining the energy and will to keep going. We call this effort "Validation." Check your weight weekly and your other targets at least monthly. Here is the instruction for an easy to use adaptable form that works very well for these other targets.

Write down your current clothes sizes and your target goals, and then follow your progress. In the "Body Dimensions" area, measure the circumference of each body area and record. Then, record your target measurements. Keep track of them on a monthly basis, especially the number of inches lost.

Clothes

	Pre-Program	Target	Mo. 1	Mo. 2	Mo. 3	Mo. 4	Mo. 5	Mo. 6
Dress								
Shirt								
Jacket								
Pants								

Body Dimensions

Neck								
Upper Arms								
Chest								
Waist								
Thighs								
Total								
Inches Lost								

% Body Fat							
BMI							

Your Thoughts:

Acquiring Energy

*"The higher your energy level, the more
efficient your body. The more efficient your
body, the better you feel and the more you
will use your talent to produce outstanding
results." Anthony Robbins*

There is no life without energy. It can be argued that
there is no good life, no happy life, and no fulfilling
life without the many different forms of energy that
fuel us. Filling our "batteries" with all the various
forms of power from all the many different available
sources is important to obtaining optimal health.

Think about the different kinds of energy you may
receive on a daily basis. How do your thoughts
compare with this list?

- Physical – food, water, and air producing
  energy from calories
- Emotional – relationships, environment, using
  gifts and talents, positive attitude, self-
  improvement, and other activities
- Spiritual – helping others, relationship with
  deity, self-improvement, finding beauty in the
  world and in people

For many of us, witnessing a beautiful day or a kind
interpersonal act fills our beings with increased vigor.

The number of ways a person can acquire energy, whether planned or at random is awe inspiring.

Why do we care? Because, your body's optimal operation or health occurs when all physiological, spiritual, and emotional factors are in balance. You want to change your life by improving your physical health and getting rid of unhealthy weight. It will take all of these forms of energy to do that.

When you get discouraged, what type of energy do you need? Some may say emotional, others spiritual, perhaps all of them, depending on what has caused the discouragement. Life's components are not easily put into little identifiable boxes. You are more complex than that.

In your quest for weight-mastery, you are going to have low energy days, perhaps low energy in each of the categories. Just because you are tired doesn't mean your goal is unworthy of your effort or is unattainable. People get tired when the fuel they need runs out. When that happens a "fill-up" is needed.

So, where do you go to get the energy you need? The need for food, water, and air is obvious. Don't focus on them right now. When your "batteries" are running low, what do you do to recharge them or who do you go to for that injection of vigor to keep you going?

You probably have some activities or people that you turn to in order to change this situation. Now is the time for you to make two lists. This first is "Activities that Give Me Energy." What do you like to do that fills your physical, emotional, and spiritual batteries? Make a complete list.

_____

_____

_____

_____

_____

_____

_____

_____

_____

_____

The second list is "People that Give Me Energy." Do the same thing and write down all the people that you can interact with for increased energy.

_____

_____

_____

_____

_____

_____

_____

_____

_____

_____

Keep these lists close by and when you feel energy draining away, go to them and find the person and/or activity that you need to restore vigor and follow through. Don't let discouragement or depression stop you from doing this. Your quest still has value and so do you.

Brain Energy

There is research that seems to indicate that when we get involved in something that is new and fills us with excitement or anticipation, the brain becomes energized by it. This energy form has an initial life of about six weeks. After that, if we are paying attention, we'll begin to recognize lowering energy levels. Don't be concerned, this is a normal pattern. It just means you need to look for help from other energy sources, as we have discussed.

Some people might interpret that this drop in energy is "intuition" that the goal and activity really isn't of value. In this case, energy depletion is a part of a biological cycle. Just because your energy level is lower does not mean the value of the activity or goal has changed. Trust yourself and the decision you made when your energy levels were higher.

This core principle is vitally important: energy is required for life, activity, thinking, fulfillment, and happiness. Become a self-advocate. Go get it from all its various healthy sources.

Fill Your Batteries from "You"

So far, we've focused on getting energy from external sources. There is an "internal" source, a reservoir of energy potential, that you should be aware of. It is the recording of your experiences and feelings. This reservoir fills as you write down what is transpiring in your life, especially your challenges and successes in your weight-mastery quest.

Just as you can draw energy from interactions with other people, you can energize yourself as you relive meeting challenges and your successes through your journal. Read what you have recorded and then visualize once again how you felt achieving your goal, no matter how small or large.

Remember, your brain can't tell the difference between a visualized and an actual experience. In this regard you have a "real" success that you are reliving, providing even greater energy potential. You will fill yourself with new vigor and strength that will keep you energized and motivated.

If you've been diligent in producing this record, you have an energy source that is readily at hand. When you feel your energy level dropping, go to your journal and read about the excitement and determination you had to succeed when you started on this pathway.

Dig into your daily thoughts, the things that you learned and your successes. There is energy magic in those pages that will keep you working and succeeding.

If you are a doubter, set that attitude aside for a while and give it a try. You may be surprised at what you can do for yourself.

Your Thoughts:

Give to Receive

"For it is in giving that we receive."St. Francis of Assisi

This chapter is about your need of support from others in order to be successful in achieving your weight-mastery and health goals. So, what does the title have to do with this? Everything!

Our client experience has made it very clear that without the help of others, few people will be successful in truly changing their brains and their lives. In fact, the generalized success expectation for any program that requires a change of habit and perspective is only about 5%. This means that only five people in 100 or one in 20 will be successful. Those are painful expectations and that is our experience in weight-mastery, unless . . .

You do things differently. Here is the X factor. When a person sets aside embarrassment, pride, fear, shyness, or any other attitude or emotion that tends to isolate her, those success numbers can be improved. Individuals are significantly more successful when they invite the participation and support of others.

Here is where the title of this chapter comes into play. For your "support" group to be successful in helping you, you must "give" or frequently share with them how you are doing. This includes successes and challenges. You'll notice that the term "failure" was not used.

So called "failures" are really only teaching opportunities to point out to you what works, what doesn't, and where you are in the process. You must "give" of yourself in this "partnership" with others in order to receive the energy and support you need to keep going and prove successful.

Arrange for Support

Every potential weight-master needs the help of some invited supporters. One of the primary reasons is that the process will likely require several months instead of a few weeks. You have already been instructed on the "six-week term" of brain energy. For a short period some people can operate alone and find success. But, longer periods usually require the help of others as regular life inserts itself in the process and energy levels and motivation may ebb and flow.

Your support team ought to be composed of a primary "Support Partner" and a secondary support group. Here are the characteristics of each.

Support Partner:

- A person who understands what you are experiencing and your desire to be successful.

- If possible, a friend or family member who is in the program with you (perhaps the best support option).
- An individual who you trust to provide continuous support while you are on this weight-mastery journey.
- This person has a copy of your self-contract and signed it along with you.
- You have a scheduled, weekly discussion about how you are doing, your successes and challenges.
- This person is a good listener and someone you can go to when you are discouraged, challenged, or excited to share a success.
- This partner won't easily let you off the hook, but will provide support, energy, and strength to keep you going. This person helps to keep your "feet to the fire" through all of life's experiences.

The Support Partner might ask any of these or other questions you decide on until fulfilled:

a. Have you identified all of your eating/food triggers?
b. Have you written your Self-Talk script(s)?
c. Have you learned your scripts?
d. Are you practicing and using your scripts daily to deal with "triggers?"

e. Are you keeping a daily journal of triggers experienced, how you handled them, challenges, and successes (including how they made you feel)?

f. Are you sharing your successes with others as they occur?

g. Have you developed and are you following a healthy eating plan?

h. Do you have an exercise plan that you are following each day?

Secondary Support Group:

- Individuals that you interact with on a frequent basis at home, work, and social occasions.

- They know what you are trying to accomplish and are supportive in their comments and interactions.

- They won't try to "test" your resolve or attempt to sabotage your efforts.

- You are comfortable performing your new, healthy behaviors in their presence and sharing with them what you are working on.

If you are surrounded by people who want you to be successful, you will find the necessary support and energy to keep going.

Volunteering

The truest form of "receiving by giving" will occur

when you volunteer to help someone else change her life as you are doing. It not only builds your self-confidence, but it proves to you that you know and practice the processes required for success. In all likelihood, you will receive far more in value than you give.

Your thoughts:

Eliminating Self-Sabotage

If you have a poor self-image, you don't really know who you are or of your inherent value.

People who do not have a good self-image have often had experiences that have left them with the deep-seated negative belief that they don't deserve to be successful or enjoy many of the good things of life.

These feelings do not have to be conscious thoughts, but nevertheless, if they reside in the subconscious mind, they will likely be acted upon. The act of sabotaging positive outcomes can become an automatic response by the subconscious mind. These sabotaged outcomes are used as "proof" by the person's mind to justify the negative beliefs he or she may have about themselves, that they are correct — even when they are not!

This may sound strange, but in light of what you have learned about brain change, this should make sense. Our brains follow scripts that have been practiced over and over.

How Does It Get Started?

Where do these negative beliefs come from? How do they get started? It may be as simple as being told as a child (by a trusted person, like a parent) that the child is stupid or unlovable, or some other negative and incorrect trait. Hearing it often enough, the person begins to internalize it and to think about herself in that way — to accept it, even though it is not true.

To personalize this, the end result is to have an internal belief that somehow you do not deserve the good things that life has to offer. So, even though you may be attracted to something that would enhance your life, your "automatic script" sabotages the effort in order to verify your negative self-conception.

What about adults? Can this happen at older ages? Yes! Do you know the feelings of rejection or fear? Have you ever lost a job? How did the loss make you feel? Perhaps you were even glad for a while, considering all the things you disliked about the work. How did you feel later, after a month, then two, then longer?

After submitting your resume many times, maybe even having a few interviews, but no job offer, how did it all make you feel? By this point in time your self-image may have begun to tarnish — you may have begun to feel that you have little value to others. What if this situation continued for a long period? Would you begin to think negative thoughts about yourself, perhaps all the time? After all, the whole world must not think much of you as evidenced by the universal lack of caring. If the whole world feels this way, then it must be true. Is it true? No, no, no!

Children and adults can develop deep negative feelings about themselves as a result of the experiences they have in life and how those experiences are perceived. The end result may very well be repeated as acts of self-sabotage, designed through long-standing negative thought and habit to confirm that negative self-appraisal.

It is important to note that we all have frustrating moments in life when we may have a poor opinion of ourselves, that's just a normal part of life. You probably have felt worthless a time or two. If negative thoughts persist, then that is a situation that should be concerning to you.

Self-Sabotaging Behaviors

The number of sabotaging behaviors a person might perform is too numerous to name. Consider this short list to determine if you have experienced thoughts or performances by you that are similar in nature and are persistent.

- Feeling that you have no value
- Distancing yourself from others
- Comparing yourself to others and always feeling you don't measure up

- Can't find a purpose for your life
- Postponing pleasure unnecessarily
- Procrastination
- Overindulging in eating or drinking
- Impulsive acts, without consideration of consequences
- Ignoring or minimizing problems
- Overly critical or judgmental of yourself
- Needing help, but not asking for it
- Difficulty in advocating or believing in yourself
- Overly fearful of possible negative results of activities or relationships (can't focus on the good possibilities)

Realistic faith and hope for the future are necessary for you to be well-adjusted, experience wellbeing, and to gain mastery of your weight and wellness. If you experience any of these behaviors on an ongoing basis, they are possible evidences of negative feelings you have about "you" and may indicate the need for you to change your beliefs and perceptions.

Is Fear a Factor?

Fear can most definitely be a factor. A person may fear not being sufficiently skilled, talented, strong, intelligent, or any other personal characteristic. That kind of judgment might have its roots in past experience or as a consequence of some kind of abuse. The net result is the formation of a negative self-concept and the likelihood of continual self-sabotage to confirm that judgment.

Fear can be a factor in the life of the person who struggles with change, dreading possible outcomes and the insecurity that might be injected into the person's life. Do you know someone who is good at their work, but continually exhibits self-sabotage when presented with opportunities for advancement, new ideas, or suggestions for improvement?

The person's subconscious may be working to keep the individual "safe" in the normal routine and situation. "What is known must be safer than the unknown." The mind's "scripting" has been developed and practiced over a long period of time to protect against the uncertainty of change.

Overcoming Self-Sabotage

Attitudes and thoughts that lead to self-sabotage are significant components of a negative brain script that may very well be an addiction. To decrease and eliminate the power of this "automatic" script and its neural pathways, the same process of Self-Talk is required. A positive script must be written and practiced that gives direction to your brain to disregard and stop protecting the incorrect perception that you are weak, and/or do not deserve good things to happen to you.

In order to develop a positive script, an understanding of what your inaccurate and negative feelings are is important. The behaviors listed above are symptoms, but not the reason your subconscious believes as it does.

What do you recall from your childhood? Have you had experiences as an adult that make you feel that you aren't as talented, capable, lovable, or valuable as others? Honesty is absolutely essential. If you recall what the cause(s) of these negative beliefs is, write it down so that it will be the focus of your script. If there is more than one cause, a script for each will be needed. If you have a negative self-image and thoughts, but can't determine the cause, a trained therapist or counselor may be needed to help you.

Self-sabotage scripts are to be written in the same manner as the others you are working on.

Here are the steps:

Step #1: Choose One Self-Sabotage Cause. Remember, the symptom or self-sabotaging behavior is usually not the cause. However, the cause, thought, and behavior are linked. If you feel you have more than one causative factor, choose the one that seems the least difficult to deal with. This will give you practice and experience for dealing with more difficult factors. For this example, the underlying cause will be, "I have been told that I am not an attractive person."

Step #2: <u>What is the triggering thought that you generally have regarding this cause?</u>

"Whenever I think about losing weight, I have the thought that it really doesn't matter, because I'm not attractive anyway."

Step #3: <u>Confronting Statement</u>.

- State the negative behavior that you habitually use (have trained your brain to use) in response to the triggering thought. "I justify not eating right or not getting some exercise, because it doesn't matter. I won't be attractive to anyone anyway."
- Describe the underlying negative belief. "My ex-husband told me for 15 years that I'm not attractive and if I divorced him, I wouldn't find anyone who wanted me."
- State the real-life consequences that result from giving in to that thought. "I don't have a good opinion of me. Every time I give into the thoughts that doing something healthy won't matter, I feel guilty for a short while. Sometimes I eat junk food to make me feel better. I am gaining weight and my clothes don't fit. I don't feel good, but the guilty feelings about having betrayed me are soon gone and I go on unable to do anything differently."

Step #4: <u>New Thought and Behavior.</u>

- State boldly and clearly the new behavior you want in place of the old one. "Whenever I have the thought that eating right or getting exercise doesn't matter, I look at the photograph of me graduating from college and say, 'This is what I will look like in a few months. I am eating healthy and getting some exercise every day.'"
- Boldly state your belief about who you are and your intrinsic values. "I am a person of value. I have talents and abilities and make a difference in the lives of others. I am good at my job and have helped our customer service department to exceed its goals in customer satisfaction. I am important to my children, coworkers, and friends."
- Describe in detail how this change in feeling about yourself makes or will make you feel. "I have never been happier in my life. I have energy and enthusiasm for life. I get up each morning excited about the new day and what I can accomplish. I love eating healthy foods and have no desire to eat junk food. I find exercising invigorating and fun, something I look forward to. My skin glows with this improved health. I have a smile on my face all day long. People wonder what I am up to and I try to tell them how happy I am. I feel fulfilled and valued every day."

Be honest in your self-appraisal regarding a negative self-image, the corresponding thoughts, and behaviors. If you have them, change them. It all begins with the way you think.

Your Thoughts:

Naturally "Thin" Attitudes

*"In order to change we must be sick and tired of
being sick and tired." Author Unknown*

Perhaps much to our frustration, there is a population
of individuals who naturally have a healthy
percentage of body fat and appropriate weight. These
people have been labeled "naturally thin." A better
description might be "naturally lean." A study of the
attitudes regarding food and the subsequent
behaviors of "naturally lean" people has great value
for those who want to copy this group and control
their weight.

There are a number of questions that seem
appropriate to ask. Do they think differently? How do
they stay lean? Do they exercise compulsively? Do
they eat certain foods? Do they control portion size?
Do they eat fast food? Do they stay away from fat? Do
they all have high metabolism? Is willpower the key
to their success?

Many researchers have studied these people in great
detail. Not surprising—a review and correlation of
their findings discloses great similarity in attitudes,
behaviors, and foods eaten among them. These people
do think differently about their bodies and about food
in general. However, their distinguishing attitudes
and behaviors can be identified, learned, and used by

you. Doing so will give you powerful tools to achieve the level of health and overall wellness you desire for the rest of your life!

Naturally Lean Mindset

Becoming a "naturally lean" person requires a change of mindset that incorporates an intuitive understanding of the value of you as a person, your body, and what it takes to keep body and mind in optimal health. This is often a total paradigm shift, linking mindset with healthy actions that become automatic.

A person can shed the attitudes and behaviors of the overweight by applying and coming to "own" the thoughts and behaviors of naturally lean people.

They regard food as a necessity to maintain life, but it is neither their "best friend" nor an object to fill emotional needs. This does not mean that they don't enjoy food; they just keep their focus on it for its real purpose — to sustain life.

1. All strategies and behaviors about food are centralized on the body's physical needs for nourishment having been met — the term we use is <u>satisfied</u>. In effect, they listen to their bodies rather than their emotions. They have an awareness of their body's real needs that

determines when eating takes place, the foods eaten, and the amounts.

2. Each bite of food provides a prompt as to how the body is responding to it. They eat slowly enough to listen and receive these prompts. When the "satisfied" signal is given, hunger pangs disappear and they stop eating, even if food is still on the plate. If a bite of food causes a negative reaction, like making the person feel sluggish, the feeling is recognized and the food is no longer consumed.

3. Scientists tell us it takes 20 minutes for the first bite of food to register with the brain. If a whole meal is eaten quickly, the hunger prompts have no value. Research has revealed that the "naturally lean" chew each bite of food 22 times on average before swallowing. In contrast, obese study subjects chewed each bite an average of four times before swallowing. Eating slowly is important to listening to your body.

4. When rewards are desired, the naturally lean often use pleasures other than food. When food is used, it is in moderation.

5. They possess optimistic and positive attitudes.

To become "naturally lean," you have to think like the "naturally lean." The attitudes and behaviors outlined here need to become second nature to you. This means you have to study and practice them. Make changing your thoughts and attitudes a part of your "self-contract" and begin to create new "attitude habits" using the Self-Talk process.

Your Thoughts:

From Thought to Action

"An active mind cannot exist in an inactive body."
General George S. Patton

Hopefully, you have understood the "brain change" processes and the power they possess to improve your life. Do you also understand a bit more about you and the innate power you have to make changes? This educational program has been designed to empower you now to go forward and change your thoughts so that your actions will produce a healthy body and long-term weight loss.

As you have learned, changing the brain is a required first step before changing the body, long-term. For many people the mental changes are more challenging than the physical. If that were not the case, we would have a much greater percentage of our population in the "healthy weight category." The "tsunami of obesity" has become our nation's most pervasive health issue and it can only be resolved one person at a time.

Here is our recommendation for a daily to-do list that will rewire your brain and help you to adopt thoughts and attitudes in tune with your weight-mastery and health goals:

- Use your "anti-goal" list as needed

- Review your self-contract
- Use creative visualization each morning
- Practice and use your Self-Talk scripts for triggers and self-sabotage as needed
- Write in your journal
- Use willpower correctly – be persistent in using the weight-mastery tools
- What self-improvement can you validate and record?
- Use your "energy activity and people lists" as needed
- Review your successes often to keep your "batteries" filled
- Work with your Support Partner as scheduled and as needed
- Interact as needed with your Support Group
- Volunteer to help others attempting to master their weight
- Think and act like a "naturally lean" person

Dual Creation – Step Two

As pointed out in the Preface, "dual creation's" **step one** is "changing your brain and thoughts." **Step two** is to begin to implement the physical processes, actions, and tools required for weight loss, long-term mastery, and optimal health.

This is now the time for you to formulate a physical plan of action for optimal health. Brain change will become the foundation for long-term success as you implement the new behaviors needed.

There are many plans and much traditional source material available for this second step. If it would be helpful for you to have a program guide that is integrated with the brain change requirements, we recommend taking a look at our "next step," the *Weight-Mastery Solution*. It is a holistic program that integrates the brain change education from this work with the physical instruction and actions needed to produce healthy weight loss and long-term mastery.

It has been written in a self-help format that is easy to follow and adapt to your specific needs. It comes with charts, tables, and other tools to simplify your efforts and make them as comprehensive and effective as possible. You will be able to follow the instruction and track your progress, all within a system that mentors you step-by-easy-to-follow-step. You'll experience why brain change must be a part of any weight loss and health program.

In addition to the brain change science, this manual/workbook includes education on the following topics and tools:

- Entrainment (self-hypnosis)
- Keeping your brain healthy
- The role of hormones
- Insulin resistance
- Nutrition guide
- Exercise and physical fitness
- Life-long plan for optimal health

- Aftercare – creating permanent change
- Specialized tools and instruction for long-term success

Whatever plan or program you decide to use, we recommend that it include the bullet point elements listed above.

Additional information on this program can be found at **www.weightmasterysolution.com**.

About the Author

Michael Steven Purles is the director of Weight-Mastery Solutions and co-developer of the *Weight-Mastery Solution* health program.

He is an author and professional trainer. In addition to *One-Day Miracles*, he has written the *Weight-Mastery Solution* and a number of manuals on business and life-skills subjects. His training assignments have taken him to many destinations throughout the United States and Canada.

Michael resides in Sandy, Utah with his wife.

Correspondence can be sent to:
info@weightmasterysolution.com